ENERGY BAR

RECIPES

Easy and Tasty Homemade Granola and
Protein Bars for Breakfast and Snack

Celeste Jarabese

TABLE OF CONTENTS

INTRODUCTION

People nowadays are always searching for quick, tasty, and healthy food that can supply the body with energy and much-needed nutrients. This is why food manufacturers around the globe are making money out of "Energy Bars," also known as Protein Bars or Granola Bars.

Energy Bars are very easy to do, so why not start making your own version at home? This way, you can say goodbye to packaged store-bought munchies that are loaded with artificial flavorings and additives. Not to mention that you can easily customize your Energy Bar as to what ingredients are available in your pantry. You can also adjust it according to your taste and health concern (if you want it gluten-free, sugar-free, Keto-friendly, Paleo-friendly, etc.).

There is no more reason to skip breakfast or snack because you can bring these power-packed bars anywhere with you. It is sure a lot of fun when you start making your own Energy Bars at home. This book will help you learn different kinds of Energy Bars, whether you are looking for baked or no-bake, chewy or crunchy recipes. Be creative because your options are truly endless! From fruits to the type of sweetener, to nuts and seeds. Just throw them all in!

These great-tasting energy bars can last for days up to a week or two when properly stored. Also, they can be easily packed and portable. You can bring them to the office, school, or at the gym for a healthy snack on the go. Sounds good, right? You bet!

So, what are you waiting for?

Let's get started!

TIPS ON MAKING THE PERFECT HOMEMADE ENERGY BARS

I've made a lot of Energy Bars over the years and have tried different sweeteners from honey to maple syrup to agave nectar to brown rice syrup. A thick syrup is needed to bind the ingredients together. I must say that the ones I've mentioned are all good, but sometimes some ingredients blend well with a particular sweetener because some have a strong flavor while others are just mild.

Agave nectar is one of the best because aside from being versatile, it is vegan and diabetic-friendly. You can use it to create both chewy bars and crunchy bars. It has a mild flavor without the bitter taste that you would typically get from common artificial sweeteners. Agave nectar is also very good at making energy bars because it is not overpowering. It lets you taste the flavor of dried fruits, nuts, and other ingredients that you are using.

When you experience that your bars don't stick together as desired, especially when you aim for chewier bars, you can add some applesauce or nut butter such as peanut butter and almond butter. Also, adding some cocoa powder mixed with agave nectar or brown rice syrup can surely do the trick in making firmer bars.

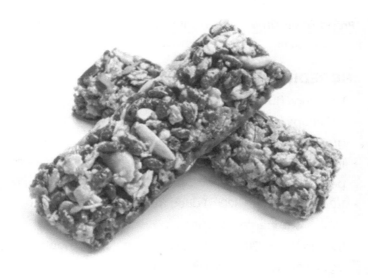

ENERGY BAR
RECIPES

HERE IS THE MOST BASIC RECIPE FOR MAKING
ENERGY BARS AT HOME. NOTES ARE ADDED
SO YOU CAN CUSTOMIZE AS DESIRED.

BASIC ENERGY BAR RECIPE

Preparation Time	Total Time	Yield
10 minutes	20 minutes	8 servings

INGREDIENTS

- 1-1/2 cups (150 g) old-fashioned oats
- 1-1/4 cups (65 g) cereal mix, or any other kind of puffed grains or cereals
- 1/2 cup (60 g) chopped nuts, such as - walnuts, almonds, pecans, or peanuts
- 1/2 - 1 cup (60 g – 120 g) dried fruits, such as – apricots, raisins, cranberries, or cherries
- 1/2 cup (160 – 170 ml) syrup, such as – honey, maple syrup, agave nectar, or brown rice syrup
- A teaspoon (5 ml) of pure vanilla extract or almond extract
- 1/4 teaspoon (1.5 g) kosher salt
- 1/2 - 1 teaspoon (1 – 2 g) spices (cinnamon, cardamom, allspice, or pumpkin pie spice)
- 3 tablespoons (45 g) peanut butter or almond butter
- 1 tablespoon (7 g) cocoa powder (optional for firmer bars)

THINGS NEEDED

- Large mixing bowl
- Spatula or Wooden spoon
- Measuring cups and spoons
- Baking pan
- Aluminum foil or Parchment paper

PROCEDURE

- Prior to Baking: Preheat and set your oven to 325 F (160 C). Put the baking rack in the middle of your oven. Line the baking pan with baking or parchment paper, leaving extra to hang over the sides. Coat lightly with oil spray. Toast both the nuts and grains for 10-15 minutes, or until toasted and fragrant. If you want to achieve softer dried fruit pieces, just soak them in very hot water for at least 10 minutes and then drain before using.
- Combining the Dry Ingredients: Mix together the oats/cereals, nuts, and dried fruits together in a mixing bowl.
- Warm the Syrup: Warm the chosen syrup for at least 10-15 seconds in a small saucepan over medium heat. It should be thick enough to be poured easily. Stir in the vanilla extract, salt, spices (if using), and nut butter (if using).
- Add the prepared Syrup into the Dry Ingredients: Pour the syrup mixture over dry ingredients. Mix until the dry ingredients are completely coated with syrup and begin to come together in clumps.
- Press mixture into the Baking Pan: Pour your energy bar mixture into the prepared pan. With a piece of wax paper, press the mixture firmly into the prepared pan (so it won't stick to your fingers and to make an even layer).
- Bake your Energy Bars: Bake your energy bars for 20-25 minutes if you want it chewy or 25-30 minutes if you want crunchy bars. Press them again with the back of a lightly oiled spatula as soon as you remove the bars from the oven. (This will give you firmer energy bars)

- Cool the Energy Bars: Let the energy bars cool completely in the baking pan. They will become firm as they cool. You can then cut into portions in the pan using a very sharp knife, then lift the energy bars by the flaps of parchment to remove from the pan. Store in between layers of wax paper in an airtight container inside the refrigerator or freezer.
- Pack them up: To make it easier to slip into backpacks and lunch boxes, you can also wrap each bar individually in foil or plastic wrap.

AMARANTH QUINOA AND WALNUT ENERGY BAR

Preparation Time	Total Time	Yield
10 minutes	40 minutes	12 servings

INGREDIENTS

- 1/2 cup (90 g) pre-washed raw quinoa
- 1/2 cup (100 g) raw amaranth
- 1 cup (100 g) walnuts
- 1 cup (125 g) mixed dried fruits
- 1/2 cup (50 g) shredded coconut, unsweetened
- 1/2 cup (160 g) agave nectar
- 2 tablespoons (40 ml) maple syrup
- 2 tablespoons (30 g) almond butter
- 1/2 teaspoon (2.5 g) salt
- 1/2 teaspoon (2.5 ml) vanilla
- cooking oil spray

PROCEDURE

- Line a 9-inch square pan with parchment paper or aluminum foil and lightly grease with oil spray. Preheat and set your oven to 350 F (175 C).
- Then, pop the quinoa and amaranth in a large pan or skillet. Set aside to cool.
- Combine the mixed fruits and walnuts to a food processor. Process in short pulses, until coarsely chopped.

- Mix together the quinoa, amaranth, shredded coconut, chopped fruits, and nuts in a medium bowl. Set aside.
- Place the agave nectar, maple syrup, almond butter, and salt in a microwave-proof bowl or measuring cup. Microwave very briefly, until just heated. Pour this mixture into the bowl with the quinoa mixture. Mix until everything is coated well.
- Transfer the energy bar mixture into the foil-lined pan. With a piece of wax paper, press the mixture firmly into the pan (so it won't stick to your fingers and so you'll have an even layer at the bottom of the pan).
- Bake mixture in the oven for about 20-25 minutes, or until it begins to turn golden brown. Take it out of the oven and allow to cool completely in the pan before cutting into portions.
- Store them in an airtight container, in between layers of wax paper, for up to one week inside the refrigerator.

NUTRITIONAL INFORMATION

Energy	Fat	Carbohydrates	Protein	Sodium
187 calories	7.7 g	27.2 g	4.9 g	102 mg

BLUEBERRY CEREAL BAR WITH YOGURT GLAZE

Preparation Time	Total Time	Yield
10 minutes	8 hours 10 minutes	12 servings

INGREDIENTS

- 2 cups (200 g) rolled oats
- 1 1/2 cup (150 g) brown rice krispies
- 1/4 cup (25 g) shredded coconut, unsweetened
- 1/4 cup (30 g) roasted almonds, coarsely chopped
- 1 1/2 tablespoons (10 g) hemp seeds
- 1/4 teaspoon (1.5 g) kosher salt
- 1/2 cup (125 g) peanut butter
- 1/2 cup (160 ml) brown rice syrup
- 1 teaspoon (5 ml) vanilla
- 1 cup (150 g) fresh blueberries

Greek Yogurt Glaze:

- 1 tablespoon (15 ml) of water
- 1 teaspoon (5 ml) vanilla extract
- 1/2 teaspoon (2.5 g) unflavored gelatin
- 1/4 cup (60 g) Greek yogurt
- 1 tablespoon (20 g) brown rice syrup
- pinch of kosher salt
- 2 cups (200 g) icing sugar

PROCEDURE

- Preheat and set your oven to 350 F (175 C). Then, line a baking sheet with a sheet of parchment paper and spread the blueberries evenly on the baking sheet.

Bake for about 30 minutes, or until the berries burst, it will also shrink. Set aside to cool.

- Line a 9 x 13 baking pan with wax or parchment paper.
- In a large bowl place the oats, rice krispies, shredded coconut, almonds, hemp seeds, and salt. Mix together.
- In a small microwave safe bowl, mix together the peanut butter and brown rice syrup. Microwave briefly, until just heated and then stir in vanilla.
- Pour the syrup mixture onto the oat mixture and mix until everything is coated well. Stir in the blueberries.
- With a piece of wax paper, press mixture firmly into the pan (so it won't stick to your fingers and to make an even layer at the bottom of the pan). Cover and freeze for about an hour. Cut into 12 bars and put it back into the freezer.
- To make the Greek yogurt glaze: Place the water and vanilla in a small bowl. Then, sprinkle with gelatin and whisk until the gelatin is evenly distributed. Set aside for about 5-7 minutes, it will set like a thick paste. In a separate small bowl, mix together the yogurt, syrup, and salt. Microwave for about 15-20 seconds or until very warm to the touch, stirring halfway through. Don't boil or the yogurt will curdle. Whisk together the gelatin and the heated yogurt mixture until the gelatin is completely dissolved. Transfer mixture into a medium mixing bowl. Beat using an electric mixer, adding the icing sugar gradually until it forms a thick, but pourable, coating.
- Line a baking sheet with parchment paper. Doing one bar at a time, gently dip the bottom of the energy bar into the yogurt mixture and let any excess to drip

off. Place on the prepared baking sheet, coated side faces up. Repeat procedure with the remaining bars. Set aside, uncovered, until dry to the touch. Transfer remaining yogurt coating in a plastic container with lid and keep in the refrigerator until ready to use again.

- Once the bars are completely dry, turn the bars over so the yogurt coated side is now facing down.
- Serve and enjoy.

NUTRITIONAL INFORMATION

Energy	Fat	Carbohydrates	Protein	Sodium
185 calories	6.6 g	28.6 g	5.1 g	100 mg

GLUTEN-FREE CARROT AND RAISIN POWER BAR

Preparation Time	Total Time	Yield
10 minutes	40 minutes	12 servings

INGREDIENTS

- 1/2 cup (50 g) coconut flour
- 1/2 cup (60 g) soy protein powder, vanilla flavor
- 1/4 cup (40 g) ground flaxseeds
- 1 teaspoon (2 g) ground cinnamon
- 1/4 teaspoon (0.5 g) ground nutmeg
- 1/4 teaspoon (0.5 g) ground cloves
- 1/4 teaspoon (1.5 g) gluten-free baking soda
- 1/4 teaspoon (1.5 g) sea salt
- 3/4 cup (85 g) shredded carrots
- 1/4 cup (30 g) seedless raisins
- 1/4 cup (80 ml) honey
- 2 tablespoon (30 g) coconut butter, melted

PROCEDURE

- Preheat and set your oven to 375 F (190 C) and line a 9 x 9-inch baking pan with foil or parchment paper. Set aside.
- Combine the coconut flour, soy protein powder, flaxseeds, spices, baking soda, and salt in a large bowl.
- Add the carrots, raisins, honey, and coconut butter. Mix until combined well. Transfer and press firmly into

the prepared baking pan.
- Bake for about 20-25 minutes, or until a toothpick inserted comes out clean. Take it out of the oven and allow to cool completely in the pan before cutting into portions.
- Serve or store in an airtight container inside the refrigerator.

NUTRITIONAL INFORMATION

Energy	Fat	Carbohydrates	Protein	Sodium
134 calories	3.8 g	16.5 g	9.3 g	83 mg

CEREAL BAR WITH CHOCOLATE CHIPS

Preparation Time	Total Time	Yield
10 minutes	35 minutes	12 servings

INGREDIENTS

- 2 cups (200 g) rolled oats
- 1 cup (100 g) chopped walnuts
- 1/2 cup (125 g) applesauce, unsweetened
- 1/2 cup (80 g) chocolate chips
- 1/2 cup (160 ml) agave nectar
- 1 teaspoon (5 ml) vanilla extract
- 1/4 tsp. (1.5 g) Kosher salt
- cooking oil spray

PROCEDURE

- Preheat and set your oven to 350 F (175 C).
- Line a 9 x 13-inch with parchment paper or aluminum foil and lightly grease with oil spray.
- Mix the oats, walnuts, applesauce, chocolate chips, agave nectar, and vanilla extract together in a large bowl.
- Press the energy bar mixture firmly into the prepared baking pan.
- Bake for about 20 minutes. Cool completely before cutting into bars.
- Serve and enjoy!

NUTRITIONAL INFORMATION

Energy	Fat	Carbohydrates	Protein	Sodium
165 calories	5.9 g	25.8 g	2.9 g	57 mg

ENERGY BAR WITH CHIA SESAME AND DATES

Preparation Time	Total Time	Yield
10 minutes	40 minutes	12 servings

INGREDIENTS

- 1 cup (100 g) rolled oats
- 1/2 cup (60 g) raw almonds
- 3/4 cup (135 g) dates, pitted
- 1/4 cup (40 g) chia seeds
- 1/4 cup (40 g) sesame seeds
- 2 tablespoons (20 g) flaxseeds
- 2 tablespoons (20 g) hemp seeds
- 1/4 cup (60 g) almond butter
- 1/4 cup (80 ml) agave nectar

PROCEDURE

- Toast your oats and almonds in a baking sheet at 350 F (175 C) oven for 12-15 minutes, or until slightly golden brown. Let cool.
- Process the oat and almond mixture in a food processor until finely ground. Transfer to a medium bowl.
- Place dates in the food processor and process for about a minute, it should form a "sticky ball".
- Add the dates and all the seeds into the bowl with ground oats and almonds. Mix well

- Warm the almond butter and agave in a small saucepan over low heat. Pour over oat mixture and then mix until coated well.
- Transfer to an 8×8-inch baking pan lined with parchment paper so they can be lifted out easily.
- Cover with parchment or plastic wrap and press it down to flatten the mixture and to prevent from being crumbly.
- Place the pan in the freezer for 20–30 minutes.
- Remove from the baking pan and cut into portions.
- Store in an airtight container for up to a week inside the refrigerator or freezer, if not eating right away.

NUTRITIONAL INFORMATION

Energy	Fat	Carbohydrates	Protein	Sodium
157 calories	7.0 g	21.1 g	4.4 g	2 mg

POWER BAR WITH STRAWBERRIES

Preparation Time	Total Time	Yield
10 minutes	40 minutes	10 servings

INGREDIENTS

- 2 tablespoons (30 ml) coconut oil
- 1/2 cup (125 g) mashed banana
- 1/3 cup (85 ml) skim milk
- 1/3 cup (110 ml) agave nectar
- 2 ½ cups (250 g) gluten-free oats
- 1 ½ cups (300 g) fresh strawberries, coarsely chopped
- cooking oil spray

PROCEDURE

- Preheat and set your oven to 300 F (150 C). Lightly grease an 8-inch square baking pan or baking dish with oil spray.
- Mix the coconut oil, mashed banana, milk, and agave nectar together in a large bowl. Stir in the oats until coated well.
- Gradually, add in the chopped strawberries. Then, press the mixture firmly into the prepared pan.
- Bake for about 20 minutes, or until golden brown. Take it out of the oven and allow to cool completely in the pan before cutting into portions.
- Cover each bar with plastic wrap, and store inside the refrigerator until ready to serve.

NUTRITIONAL INFORMATION

Energy	Fat	Carbohydrates	Protein	Sodium
126 calories	3.4 g	22.2 g	2.6 g	5 mg

RAW VEGAN ENERGY BAR WITH CACAO

Preparation Time	Total Time	Yield
10 minutes	1 hour 30 minutes	16 servings

INGREDIENTS

- 1 cup (100 g) walnuts
- 3/4 cup (100 g) pumpkin seeds
- 1/3 cup (60 g) ground flaxseeds
- 1/3 cup (60 g) chia seeds
- 1/3 cup (60 g) hemp seeds
- 1/4 cup (25 g) coconut flakes
- 1/4 cup (30 g) cacao nibs
- 1 cup (180 g) dates, pitted
- 1/2 cup (60 g) seedless raisins
- 3 tablespoons (45 ml) coconut oil

PROCEDURE

- Grease and line with wax or parchment paper an 8-inch square baking pan.
- Combine all dry ingredients in a food processor, leaving a little bit of each ingredient to be added later as topping.
- Add the dates and raisins into the food processor and process until everything starts to come together. If it becomes too dry, just add more coconut oil. Press this mixture and the reserved ingredients into a lined pan and place in the refrigerator to set for at least 2 hours.
- Cut into portions and store for up to one week in an

airtight container inside the refrigerator.

• Serve and enjoy!

Optional:

• You can also top it with some chocolate chips and nuts if desired.

NUTRITIONAL INFORMATION

Energy	Fat	Carbohydrates	Protein	Sodium
198 calories	13.3 g	17.5 g	5.1 g	3 mg

FRUIT AND NUT CEREAL BAR

Preparation Time	Total Time	Yield
10 minutes	40 minutes	16 servings

INGREDIENTS

- 2 cups (200 g) old-fashioned oats
- 1/2 cup (125 g) peanut butter
- 2 tablespoons (30 ml) coconut oil
- 1/2 cup (160 g) brown rice syrup
- 1 teaspoon (2 g) ground cinnamon
- 1 teaspoon (5 ml) pure vanilla extract
- 3/4 cup (90 g) almonds, coarsely chopped
- 3/4 cup (90 g) hazelnuts, coarsely chopped
- 1/2 cup (60 g) dried cherries
- 1/2 cup (60 g) raisins
- cooking oil spray

PROCEDURE

- Preheat and set your oven to 300 F (150 C). Line a 9 x 13-inch baking pan with parchment paper or aluminum foil and lightly grease with oil spray
- In a small saucepan over medium-low flame, heat the coconut oil and then stir in peanut butter until combined well.
- Add the brown rice syrup, cinnamon, and vanilla. Mix well and remove from heat.
- In a heat-proof glass bowl, mix together the oats, nuts, and dried fruits.

- Stir in peanut butter mixture until coated well.
- Transfer the mixture into the prepared baking pan and spread out the mixture evenly. Using a parchment paper press it down to make firm bars.
- Bake for 20-25 minutes. Take it out of the oven and allow to cool completely in the pan before cutting into portions.
- Serve or store in an airtight container.

NUTRITIONAL INFORMATION

Energy	Fat	Carbohydrates	Protein	Sodium
208 calories	10.9 g	25.4 g	5.3 g	45 mg

EASY GRANOLA BAR

Preparation Time	Total Time	Yield
10 minutes	40 minutes	12 servings

INGREDIENTS

- 1 cup (100 g) old-fashioned oats
- 1 cup (100 g) walnuts
- 1/2 cup (60 g) dried raisins
- 1/2 cup (60 g) dried apricots
- 1/2 cup (160 ml) agave nectar
- 2 tablespoons (30 g) applesauce, unsweetened (or add more if needed)
- 1/2 teaspoon (2.5 g) kosher salt
- 1 teaspoon (5 ml) pure vanilla extract
- cooking oil spray

PROCEDURE

- Get a 9-inch square pan and line with parchment paper or aluminum foil. Lightly grease with oil spray. Preheat and set your oven to 325 F (160 C).
- Combine the walnuts and dried fruits to a food processor. Process in short pulses, until coarsely chopped.
- Mix together the oats, walnuts, and chopped fruits in a large bowl.
- Stir in agave nectar, applesauce, salt, and vanilla until coated well.
- With a piece of wax paper, press the mixture firmly into the pan (so it won't stick to your fingers and to make an even layer at the bottom of the pan).

- Bake for about 20-25 minutes, or until it begins to turn golden brown. Take it out of the oven and allow to cool completely in the pan before cutting into portions.
- Store them in an airtight container, in between layers of parchment paper, for up to one week inside the refrigerator.

NUTRITIONAL INFORMATION

Energy	Fat	Carbohydrates	Protein	Sodium
140 calories	6.5 g	19.8 g	3.2 g	98 mg

CHOCOLATE COATED ENERGY BAR

Preparation Time	Total Time	Yield
15 minutes	45 minutes	12 servings

INGREDIENTS

- 2 cups (200 g) old-fashioned oats
- 1-1/2 cup (150 g) brown rice krispies
- 1/4 cup (25 g) shredded coconut, unsweetened
- 1/4 cup (25 g) roasted pecans, coarsely chopped
- 1-1/2 tablespoons (15 g) flaxseeds
- 1/4 teaspoon (1.5 g) kosher salt
- 1/2 cup (125 g) almond butter
- 1/2 cup (160 ml) agave nectar
- 1/2 teaspoon (5 ml) pure vanilla extract
- cooking oil spray

Chocolate Coating:

- 2 tablespoons (30 ml) of coconut oil
- 4 oz. (120 g) semisweet chocolate, chopped
- 2 tablespoons (40 ml) agave nectar
- 1/2 teaspoon (2.5 ml) vanilla extract
- pinch of kosher salt

PROCEDURE

- Line a 9 x 13 baking pan with wax or parchment paper and spray lightly with oil.
- In a large bowl place the oats, rice krispies, shredded coconut, pecans, flaxseeds, and salt. Mix together.
- In a small microwave safe bowl, mix together the almond butter and agave nectar. Microwave briefly,

until just heated and then stir in vanilla.

- Pour the almond butter mixture to the oat mixture and mix until everything is coated well.
- With a piece of wax paper, press the mixture firmly into the pan (so it won't stick to your fingers and to make an even layer at the bottom of the pan). Cover and freeze for about an hour. Cut into 12 bars and put it back into the freezer.
- To make the Chocolate coating: Heat oil in a small saucepan over medium-low heat. Add the chocolate, agave nectar, vanilla extract, and salt. Mix well until it forms a thick, but pourable, coating.
- Line a baking sheet with parchment paper. Doing one bar at a time, gently dip the bottom of the energy bar into the chocolate coating mixture and let any excess to drip off. Place on the prepared baking sheet, coated side faces up. Repeat procedure with the remaining bars. Set aside, uncovered, until dry to the touch. Transfer remaining chocolate coating in a plastic container with lid and set aside until ready to use again.
- Once the bars are completely dry, turn the bars over so the chocolate coated side is now facing down. Drizzle with remaining chocolate coating.
- Serve and enjoy!

NUTRITIONAL INFORMATION

Energy	Fat	Carbohydrates	Protein	Sodium
159 calories	10.4 g	18.0 g	2.2 g	52 mg

POWER-PACKED CEREAL BAR

Preparation Time	Total Time	Yield
10 minutes	20 minutes	12 servings

INGREDIENTS

Homemade Date Paste

- 2 cups (360 g) pitted Medjool dates
- 1/2 cup (125 ml) water

Granola Bars

- 1/2 cup (125 g) creamy peanut butter, unsalted
- 1/4 cup (60 ml) coconut oil
- 1 teaspoon (5 ml) pure vanilla extract
- 1/2 cup (100 g) almond flour
- 1/2 cup (100 g) shredded coconut, unsweetened
- 1 teaspoon (3.5 g) ground flaxseeds
- 1/2 teaspoon (1 g) ground cinnamon
- 1/4 teaspoon (0.5 g) nutmeg
- 1/4 teaspoon (1.5 g) kosher salt
- 1-3/4 cups (175 g) old-fashioned oats, toasted
- 1/4 cup (30 g) raw almonds, divided
- 1/4 cup (30 g) dried cranberries, divided
- 2 tablespoons (20 g) sunflower seeds
- 2 tablespoons (20 g) pumpkin seeds
- cooking oil spray

PROCEDURE

- Line a 9 x 13-inch baking pan with parchment paper or foil that has been sprayed lightly with oil spray leaving an overhang on the sides of the pan for easy removal.
- Combine dates and water to a medium saucepan and cook on medium low heat. Using a fork, stir and

mash the dates as the mixture heats up. The dates will soften after about 5 minutes. Continue stirring and mashing until it forms a thick paste, it is fine to have some bits.

- Add the peanut butter and coconut oil to the saucepan. Stir well to combine. Turn off heat. Stir in vanilla extract.
- Gradually, add the almond flour, shredded coconut, ground cinnamon, nutmeg and salt.
- Add in the oats, almonds, cranberries, sunflower seeds, and pumpkin seeds. Mix until coated well.
- Transfer into the prepared pan. Press using a sheet of parchment paper to make a firm and even layer. Refrigerate or freeze to harden before cutting into portions.
- Serve or store in airtight container inside the refrigerator for up to one week.

NUTRITIONAL INFORMATION

Energy	Fat	Carbohydrates	Protein	Sodium
189 calories	13.2 g	16.7 g	3.5 g	63 mg

STRAWBERRY NUT BARS

Preparation Time	Total Time	Yield
10 minutes	40 minutes	8 servings

INGREDIENTS

- 3 cups (600 g) strawberries
- 3 Tbsp. (45 ml) coconut oil
- 1/4 cup (80 ml) honey
- 1 teaspoon (5 ml) vanilla, optional
- 2 cups (200 g) rolled oats
- 1/4 teaspoon (1.5 g) salt
- 1/2 cup (90 g) pitted dates, chopped
- 1/2 cup (50 g) walnuts, chopped
- cooking oil spray

PROCEDURE

- Preheat and set your oven to 350 F (175 C). Lightly grease a 9 x 9-inch baking dish or pan with oil spray.
- Place 2 cups of strawberries in a food processor. Process until liquefied; transfer to a bowl. Stir in honey and vanilla. Then, add in the oats, salt, dates, and walnuts.
- Pulse the remaining strawberries until coarsely chopped and add into the mixture.
- Press the mixture evenly into the prepared baking pan.
- Bake for 25-30 minutes or until the edges just begin to crisp up.
- Place the baking pan on a wire rack to cool completely

before cutting into bars.

- Store leftover bars in an airtight container inside the refrigerator for up to one week.

NUTRITIONAL INFORMATION

Energy	Fat	Carbohydrates	Protein	Sodium
168 calories	7.5 g	24.0 g	3.5 g	52 mg

GRANOLA WITH RASPBERRY AND PECAN

Preparation Time	Total Time	Yield
10 minutes	40 minutes	10 servings

INGREDIENTS

- 1-1/4 cup (125 g) pecan nuts, coarsely chopped
- 1-1/2 cups (150 g) old-fashioned rolled oats
- 1/4 cup (80 ml) brown rice syrup
- 1/4 cup (60 g) applesauce, unsweetened
- 1/2 cup (125 g) raspberry preserves
- 1/4 teaspoon (1.5 g) kosher salt
- cooking oil spray

PROCEDURE

- Line a 9-inch square pan with parchment paper or aluminum foil and lightly grease with oil spray. Preheat and set the oven to 350 F (175 C).
- Mix together the brown rice syrup, applesauce, raspberry preserves, and salt in a large bowl.
- Add the pecans and rolled oats. Mix until coated well.
- With a piece of wax paper, press mixture firmly onto the pan (so it won't stick to your fingers and to make an even layer at the bottom of the pan).
- Bake mixture in the oven for about 20-25 minutes, or until it begins to turn golden brown. Take it out of the oven and allow to cool completely in the pan before cutting into portions.
- Store them in an airtight container, in between layers

of parchment paper, for up to one week inside the refrigerator.

NUTRITIONAL INFORMATION

Energy	Fat	Carbohydrates	Protein	Sodium
164 calories	8.8 g	21.2 g	1.7 g	64 mg

STRAWBERRY FILLED ENERGY BARS

Preparation Time	Total Time	Yield
10 minutes	55 minutes	16 servings

INGREDIENTS

- 2 cups (200 g) almond flour
- 1-1/2 cups (150 g) old-fashioned rolled oats, finely ground
- 1/2 teaspoon (2.5 g) kosher salt
- 1/2 teaspoon (3 g) baking soda
- 2/3 cup (220 ml) maple syrup
- 2/3 cup (165 g) unsalted butter, melted, plus more for greasing the pan
- 1 cup (250 g) strawberry preserves

PROCEDURE

- Preheat and set your oven to 350 F (175 C). Lightly grease an 8-inch square baking pan with butter and line the bottom and sides with baking paper.
- Mix together the almond flour with the ground oats, salt, and baking soda in a large bowl.
- With a wooden spoon, stir in the maple syrup and melted butter until the oat mixture is thoroughly combined.
- Press half of the oat mixture to make an even layer on the bottom of the prepared baking pan and spread the strawberry preserves on top. Then, add the remaining oat mixture to cover the filling.
- Bake the bars for about 40-45 minutes, turning the

pan halfway through baking process, until golden brown.

- Transfer to a wire rack and let the energy bars to cool completely before you take out from the pan and cut into portions.
- Serve or store in airtight containers inside the refrigerator for up to one week.

NUTRITIONAL INFORMATION

Energy	Fat	Carbohydrates	Protein	Sodium
180 calories	9.9 g	21.5 g	1.8 g	172 mg

ENERGY BAR WITH CRANBERRY AND APRICOT

Preparation Time	Total Time	Yield
10 minutes	40 minutes	12 servings

INGREDIENTS

- 2 cups (200 g) rolled oats
- 1/2 cup (50 g) wheat germ
- 1 teaspoon (2 g) ground cinnamon
- 1 cup (100 g) almond meal
- 1/3 cup (40 g) dried cranberries
- 1/3 cup (40 g) dried apricots
- 1/2 teaspoon (1.5 g) salt
- 1/2 cup (160 ml) agave nectar
- 1/2 cup (170 ml) honey
- 1 (60 g) whole egg, lightly beaten
- 1/2 cup (125 g) applesauce, unsweetened
- 1 teaspoon (5 ml) pure vanilla extract
- cooking oil spray

PROCEDURE

- Preheat and set your oven to 350 F (175 C). Grease lightly a 9 x 13-inch baking pan with oil spray and then line with foil or parchment paper.
- Mix together the oats, wheat germ, cinnamon, almond meal, cranberries, apricots, and salt in a large bowl. Create a well in the center, and pour in the agave

nectar, honey, egg, applesauce, and vanilla extract. Mix until combined well.

- Using a small sheet of parchment paper, press the mixture evenly into the baking pan.
- Bake for about 25-30 minutes in the oven, or until the bars begin to turn golden brown. Take it out of the oven and allow to cool completely in the pan before cutting into portions.
- Serve or store in airtight containers inside the refrigerator for up to one week.

NUTRITIONAL INFORMATION

Energy	Fat	Carbohydrates	Protein	Sodium
160 calories	4.3 g	28.2 g	4.1 g	114 mg

MUESLI BAR WITH CHOCOLATE CHIPS AND ALMONDS

Preparation Time	Total Time	Yield
10 minutes	40 minutes	10 servings

INGREDIENTS

- 2/3 cup (165 ml) almond milk, unsweetened
- 1/4 cup (80 ml) agave nectar
- 1 medium (120 g) ripe banana, mashed
- 2-1/2 tablespoons (25 g) chia seeds
- 1/2 teaspoon (1 g) ground cinnamon
- 1-1/2 cups (75 g) dry Muesli
- 1/4 cup (30 g) almonds, roughly chopped
- 1/4 cup (40 g) semisweet chocolate chips
- cooking oil spray

PROCEDURE

- Preheat and set your oven to 350 F (175 C).
- Mix together the first 4 ingredients in a large bowl until combined well. Set aside.
- Add the remaining dry ingredients in a separate bowl. When evenly mixed, gradually add dry ingredients into the bowl with wet mixture, making sure everything gets evenly coated. If mixture looks too wet, feel free to add more Muesli.
- Ideally, you will use a 9 x 9-inch pan to make these bars. Spray your pan with oil and line with baking

paper with overhang on the sides.

- Press the mixture firmly into the pan.
- Bake for 20-25 minutes. Take it out of the oven and allow to cool completely in the pan before cutting into portions.
- Serve or keep in an airtight container. Alternatively, you can wrap the bars individually and keep in the fridge for up to one week.

NUTRITIONAL INFORMATION

Energy	Fat	Carbohydrates	Protein	Sodium
130 calories	4.7 g	21.3 g	2.1 g	37 mg

GRANOLA BAR WITH DRIED FRUITS

Preparation Time	Total Time	Yield
10 minutes	40 minutes	16 servings

INGREDIENTS

- 2 cups (200 g) old-fashioned oats
- 1 cup (30 g) rice krispies
- 2/3 cup (80 g) dried cherries
- 1/3 cup (40 g) dried apricots
- 1/2 cup (50 g) wheat germ
- 1/2 teaspoon (1.5 g) salt
- 1/2 teaspoon (1 g) ground cinnamon
- 1/2 cup (50 g) walnuts, chopped
- 2/3 cup (225 ml) honey
- 1/2 cup (160 ml) agave nectar
- 1/2 cup (125 g) applesauce, unsweetened
- 2 tablespoons (30 ml) coconut oil
- 1 teaspoon (5 ml) vanilla extract
- cooking oil spray

PROCEDURE

- Preheat and set your oven to 350 F (175 C). Line a 9 x 13 inch baking pan with foil or baking paper, and grease with oil spray.
- In a large bowl, stir together oats, rice krispies, dried fruits, wheat germ, salt, cinnamon, and chopped walnuts.
- In a medium bowl, combine the honey, agave nectar,

applesauce, coconut oil, and vanilla extract. Pour this mixture into the dry ingredients. Mix until coated well.

- Press evenly into the prepared baking pan.
- Bake in the oven for about 25 to 30 minutes, or until the edges begin to turn golden. Take it out of the oven and allow to cool completely in the pan before cutting into portions.
- Serve or place in an airtight container. Alternatively, you can wrap the bars and keep in the fridge for up to one week.

NUTRITIONAL INFORMATION

Energy	Fat	Carbohydrates	Protein	Sodium
167 calories	4.6 g	31.0 g	2.3 g	86 mg

CHEWY ENERGY BAR WITH CHOCOLATE

Preparation Time	Total Time	Yield
10 minutes	40 minutes	16 servings

INGREDIENTS

- 1/2 cup (110 g) packed brown sugar
- 2/3 cup (165 g) peanut butter
- 1/3 cup (105 ml) agave nectar
- 1/2 cup (125 g) applesauce, unsweetened
- 1-½ teaspoons (7.5 ml) vanilla extract
- 3 cups (300 g) old-fashioned rolled oats
- 2/3 cup (105 g) chocolate chips
- 2/3 cup (70 g) walnuts, coarsely chopped
- 2/3 cup (70 g) wheat germ
- cooking oil spray

PROCEDURE

- Preheat and set your oven to 350 F (175 C). Grease a 9 x 13-inch baking pan with oil spray and line with baking paper or foil.
- In a small saucepan over medium-low heat, stir together the brown sugar, peanut butter, agave nectar, applesauce, and vanilla extract until sugar is dissolved.
- In a large bowl, stir together the oats, chocolate chips, walnuts, and wheat germ.
- Gradually, pour the peanut butter mixture into the dry mixture until coated well. Then, press lightly into the

prepared pan.
- Bake for about 20-25 minutes in the oven, or until slightly golden. Take it out of the oven and allow to cool completely in the pan before cutting into portions.
- Serve or place in an airtight container. Alternatively, you can wrap the bars and keep in the fridge for up to one week.

NUTRITIONAL INFORMATION

Energy	Fat	Carbohydrates	Protein	Sodium
183 calories	9.4 g	21.5 g	5.2 g	43 mg

GRANOLA BAR WITH POMEGRANATE

Preparation Time	Total Time	Yield
10 minutes	40 minutes	12 servings

INGREDIENTS

- 1/2 cup (125 g) applesauce, unsweetened
- 2/3 cup (215 ml) brown rice syrup
- 2 tablespoons (30 g) butter, melted
- 1-1/4 cups (125 g) quick cooking oats
- 1/3 cup (35 g) shredded coconut
- 1/3 cup (40 g) chopped almonds
- 2 tablespoons (20 g) sesame seeds
- 1/2 cup (125 g) pomegranate preserves
- 1/4 cup (30 g) seedless raisins
- 1/4 cup (30 g) dried apricots
- cooking oil spray

PROCEDURE

- Preheat and set your oven to 350 F. Grease one 9 x 13 inch square pan with oil spray and line with parchment paper.
- In a large bowl, combine the applesauce, syrup, butter, and pomegranate preserves until blended well.
- In a separate bowl, mix together the oats, coconut, almonds, sesame seeds, raisins, and dried apricots.
- Gradually, stir in dry mixture into the wet mixture until everything is coated well.
- Press mixture into the bottom of the prepared pan.

Bake for 20-25 minutes, or until golden. Take it out of the oven and allow to cool completely in the pan before cutting into portions.

- Serve or place in an airtight container. Alternatively, you can wrap the bars and keep in the fridge for up to one week.

NUTRITIONAL INFORMATION

Energy	Fat	Carbohydrates	Protein	Sodium
180 calories	6.5 g	29.7 g	2.3 g	25 mg

FRUITY ENERGY BAR WITH SESAME

Preparation Time	Total Time	Yield
10 minutes	40 minutes	20 servings

INGREDIENTS

- 3/4 cup (240 ml) brown rice syrup
- 1/2 cup (170 ml) honey
- 1/2 cup (125 g) butter, melted
- 1/4 cup (60 ml) water
- 1/2 teaspoon (2.5 g) salt
- 3 cups (300 g) rolled oats
- 1 cup (125 g) toasted and sliced almonds
- 3/4 cup (75 g) wheat germ
- 1/4 cup (40 g) pumpkin seeds
- 1/4 cup (40 g) sesame seeds
- 1/2 cup (60 g) dried cherries
- 1/2 cup (60 g) raisins
- 1/2 cup (90 g) chopped pitted dates

PROCEDURE

- In a large saucepan, combine the brown rice syrup, honey, butter, water, and salt. Simmer for 5-7 minutes over medium-low flame.
- Stir in oats, almonds, wheat germ, pumpkin seeds, and sesame seeds. Cook for 15 minutes, stirring frequently. Remove from heat and add the fruits. Mix until everything is well coated.
- Pour mixture evenly into a jelly roll pan lined with foil or

parchment paper.
- Score deeply to make bars. Allow to cool completely in the pan. Cut along the score lines.
- Serve or store in an airtight container.

NUTRITIONAL INFORMATION

Energy	Fat	Carbohydrates	Protein	Sodium
177 calories	8.8 g	23.9 g	3.1 g	93 mg

ENERGY BAR WITH DRIED CRANBERRIES

Preparation Time	Total Time	Yield
10 minutes	40 minutes	12 servings

INGREDIENTS

- 2 cups (200 g) rolled oats
- 1/2 cup (60 g) dried cranberries
- 1/2 cup (60 g) cashew nuts, coarsely chopped
- 1 1/2 teaspoons (3 g) ground cardamom
- 4 tablespoons (60 ml) coconut oil
- 1/3 cup (75 g) brown rice syrup
- 1/3 cup (115 ml) honey
- cooking oil spray

PROCEDURE

- Preheat and set your oven to 350 F (175 C).
- Line a 9-inch square pan with foil, with some extension over the sides. Grease the foil lightly with oil spray.
- Mix together the first 4 ingredients in a large bowl.
- Heat the coconut oil, brown rice syrup, and honey in a saucepan until the mixture starts to boil.
- Pour this mixture over the dry ingredients. Mix until well-coated.
- Press into the prepared pan using a spatula.
- Bake about 25-30 minutes or until the top is slightly golden brown. Take it out of the oven and allow to cool completely in the pan before cutting into portions.
- Serve or store in an airtight container.

NUTRITIONAL INFORMATION

Energy	Fat	Carbohydrates	Protein	Sodium
192 calories	8.1 g	29.5 g	2.8 g	3 mg

EASY ENERGY BAR WITH HONEY

Preparation Time	Total Time	Yield
20 minutes	40 minutes	12 servings

INGREDIENTS

- 1 cup (30 g) cornflakes
- 1/2 cup (15 g) rice krispies
- 1/2 cup (50 g) walnuts, coarsely chopped
- 1 cup (125 g) mixed dried fruits, coarsely chopped
- 1/2 cup (50 g) shredded coconut
- 2/3 cup (225 ml) honey
- 2 tablespoons (30 g) almond butter
- 1/2 teaspoon (2.5 g) salt
- 1/2 teaspoon (2.5 ml) vanilla
- cooking oil spray

PROCEDURE

- Preheat and set your oven to 350 F (175 C). Grease lightly a 9-inch square baking pan with oil spray and line with parchment paper.
- Mix together the cornflakes, rice krispies, walnuts, dried fruits, and shredded coconut to a medium bowl. Set aside.
- Place the honey, almond butter, salt, and vanilla in a microwave-safe bowl or measuring cup. Microwave very briefly, until just heated. Pour this mixture into the bowl with the quinoa mixture. Mix until everything is coated well.

- With a piece of wax paper, press mixture firmly into the pan (so it won't stick to your fingers and to make an even layer at the bottom of the pan).
- Bake in the oven for about 15–20 minutes. Take it out of the oven and allow to cool completely in the pan before cutting into portions.
- Store them in an airtight container, for up to one week inside the refrigerator.

NUTRITIONAL INFORMATION

Energy	Fat	Carbohydrates	Protein	Sodium
161 calories	5.7 g	27.9 g	2.5 g	125 mg

ALMOND AND DATE GRANOLA BAR

Preparation Time	Total Time	Yield
15 minutes	1 hour	16 servings

INGREDIENTS

- 2/3 cup (165 g) almond butter
- 1/2 cup (125 ml) skim milk
- 1/3 cup (85 g) applesauce, unsweetened
- 1/3 cup (110 ml) agave nectar
- 3 cups (300 g) old-fashioned rolled oats
- 1 cup (180 g) dates, pitted and coarsely chopped
- 1 cup (125 g) dry roasted almonds, coarsely chopped
- 2 teaspoons (4 g) ground cinnamon
- 1/2 teaspoon (1 g) ground nutmeg
- 1 teaspoon (6 g) baking soda

PROCEDURE

- Preheat and set your oven to 350 F (175 C). Grease lightly a 9 x 13-inch baking dish with oil spray and line with parchment paper.
- Mix together the almond butter, milk, applesauce, and agave nectar in a small saucepan. Cook, stirring over medium-low flame until just heated through.
- Combine the oats, dates, almonds, cinnamon, nutmeg, and baking soda in a large bowl, until evenly distributed.
- Gradually, pour in the wet mixture. Mix until coated well.

- Spread mixture into the prepared baking dish. Press with spatula to have firm bars.
- Bake in the preheated oven for about 25 to 30 minutes. Let the granola cool completely in the pan before cutting into bars.
- Serve or store in an airtight container.

NUTRITIONAL INFORMATION

Energy	Fat	Carbohydrates	Protein	Sodium
164 calories	5.3 g	28.1 g	3.9 g	110 mg

NO-BAKE APRICOT AND SULTANA PROTEIN BARS

Preparation Time	Total Time	Yield
10 minutes	40 minutes	10 servings

INGREDIENTS

- 1/2 cup (50 g) old-fashioned oats, toasted
- 1/4 cup (40 g) sunflower seeds
- 1/4 cup (30 g) dried apricots, chopped
- 1/4 cup (30 g) sultanas
- 1/4 cup (30 g) sliced almonds
- 1/4 cup (40 g) hemp seeds
- 1/4 cup (30 g) protein powder
- 1/4 cup (80 ml) agave nectar
- 1/4 cup (60 g) almond butter
- 1 tablespoon (15 ml) extra-virgin olive oil, or as needed

PROCEDURE

- Combine the oats, sunflower seeds, apricots, sultanas, almonds, hemp seed, and protein powder in a large bowl. Mix well.
- Stir in agave nectar, almond butter, and olive oil until well combined.
- Press the mixture firmly into a lightly greased 8 x 8-inch baking pan lined with wax or baking paper. Cover with plastic wrap and chill for at least 2 hours before cutting into bars.

- Serve or store in an airtight container.

NUTRITIONAL INFORMATION

Energy	Fat	Carbohydrates	Protein	Sodium
172 calories	7.3 g	14.1 g	13.9 g	112 mg

ALMOND OAT AND RAISIN ENERGY BAR

Preparation Time	Total Time	Yield
10 minutes	40 minutes	12 servings

INGREDIENTS

- 1 cup (250 g) almond butter
- 1/2 cup (170 ml) honey
- 1-1/4 cups (125 g) rolled oats, ground
- 1/2 cup (60 g) raisins
- 1/4 cup (40 g) sesame seeds
- 1/4 cup (25 g) shredded coconut, unsweetened
- 1/4 cup (25 g) walnuts, finely chopped
- 1/4 cup (40 g) ground flax seeds
- 1/4 cup (40 g) hemp seeds
- pinch of kosher salt, or to taste
- cooking oil spray

PROCEDURE

- Preheat and set your oven to 350 F (175 C). Grease a 9 x 13-inch baking pan with oil spray and line with baking paper.
- In a small saucepan, melt the almond butter. Then, stir in honey and mix until smooth.
- Place the oats, raisins, sesame seeds, shredded coconut, walnuts, flaxseeds, hemp seeds, and salt in a large mixing bowl.
- Stir in wet mixture. Mix until coated well.
- Press the oat mixture into the prepared baking pan to

make firm bars.

- Bake for 20-25 minutes. Take it out of the oven and allow to cool completely in the pan before cutting into portions.
- Serve or store in an airtight container.

NUTRITIONAL INFORMATION

Energy	Fat	Carbohydrates	Protein	Sodium
187 calories	9.0 g	23.9 g	5.2 g	3 mg

PEANUT BUTTER ENERGY BARS

Preparation Time	Total Time	Yield
15 minutes	40 minutes	12 servings

INGREDIENTS

- 3/4 cup (185 g) peanut butter
- 1/2 cup (160 ml) agave nectar
- 1-1/4 cups (125 g) old-fashioned rolled oats, ground
- 1/4 cup (30 g) sultanas
- 1/4 cup (25 g) wheat germ
- 1/4 cup (25 g) shredded coconut, unsweetened
- 1/4 cup (40 g) dry roasted peanuts, chopped
- 1/4 cup (30 g) dried cherries, chopped
- 2 tablespoons (20 g) ground flaxseeds
- 2 tablespoons (20 g) chia seeds
- pinch of kosher salt
- cooking oil spray

PROCEDURE

- Preheat and set your oven to 350 F (175 C). Grease a 9 x 13-inch baking pan with oil spray and line with baking paper.
- In a microwave-safe bowl, microwave the peanut butter until softened, about 30-35 seconds. Stir in agave nectar and mix until smooth.
- Place the oats, sultanas, wheat germ, shredded coconut, peanuts, dried cherries, flaxseeds, chia seeds, and salt. Mix until coated well.

- Press mixture into the prepared baking pan to make firm bars.
- Bake for 20–25 minutes. Take it out of the oven and allow to cool completely in the pan before cutting into portions.
- Serve or store in an airtight container.

NUTRITIONAL INFORMATION

Energy	Fat	Carbohydrates	Protein	Sodium
181 calories	10.4 g	18.4 g	6.0 g	67 mg

NUTTY ENERGY BARS WITH SUNFLOWER SEEDS

Preparation Time	Total Time	Yield
10 minutes	40 minutes	16 servings

INGREDIENTS

- 1 cup (100 g) rolled oats
- 1 cup (100 g) unsweetened coconut flakes
- 1/2 cup (50 g) wheat germ
- 1/2 cup (80 g) sesame seeds
- 1/2 cup (80 g) sunflower kernels
- 1/2 cup (80 g) pumpkin seeds
- 1 cup (125 g) sultanas
- 1/2 cup (125 g) applesauce
- 1/2 cup (160 ml) maple syrup
- 1/3 cup (75 g) brown sugar

PROCEDURE

- Grease and line a 9 x 13-inch baking pan with wax or baking paper.
- In a large frying pan, cook the oats, coconut flakes, wheat germ, sesame seeds, sunflower kernels, and pumpkin seeds over medium heat, stirring frequently, for about 8 to 10 minutes. Transfer to a large bowl. Stir in the sultanas and set aside to cool.
- In a small saucepan, heat applesauce, maple syrup, and brown sugar over medium flame; stirring

frequently, for 3 to 5 minutes or until sugar is dissolved. Pour this mixture into the dry ingredients. Mix until everything is coated well.

- Transfer mixture into the prepared pan. Using a large metal spoon or a spatula to press down firmly.
- Let it cool to room temperature then cover and chill for at least 2 hours before cutting into bars.
- Serve or store in an airtight container for up to 7 days inside the refrigerator.

NUTRITIONAL INFORMATION

Energy	Fat	Carbohydrates	Protein	Sodium
179 calories	9.3 g	21.7 g	4.4 g	6 mg

MIXED FRUIT MUESLI BAR

Preparation Time	Total Time	Yield
10 minutes	30 minutes	12 servings

INGREDIENTS

- 1-1/2 cups (150 g) almond meal
- 1-1/4 cups (65 g) toasted muesli
- 2/3 cup (80 g) dry roasted almonds, chopped
- 1/2 cup (90 g) Medjool dates, pitted, chopped
- 1/2 cup (90 g) pitted prunes, chopped
- 1/3 cup (40 g) dried currants, chopped
- 1/3 cup (40 g) dried cranberries, chopped
- 1/2 cup (80 g) sunflower seeds
- 2 tablespoons (20 g) linseed
- 2 tablespoons (7 g) raw cacao powder
- 2 teaspoons (4 g) ground cinnamon
- 2 tablespoons (30 g) tahini
- 1/2 cup (170 ml) honey
- 1/3 cup (85 ml) orange juice

PROCEDURE

- Grease and line the base and sides of a 9 x 13-inch cake pan with wax or baking paper.
- Mix together all the dry ingredients in a large bowl, reserving muesli.
- In another bowl, combine the tahini, honey, and orange juice. Mix well. Pour this mixture into the dry ingredients; stir to combine. You can add more juice

if mixture is dry.

- Transfer mixture into the prepared pan, sprinkle over remaining muesli, then press to make firm bars. Cover with plastic wrap and chill for a couple of hours before cutting into bars.
- Serve and enjoy!

NUTRITIONAL INFORMATION

Energy	Fat	Carbohydrates	Protein	Sodium
181 calories	9.1 g	23.0 g	4.5 g	6 mg

POWER BAR WITH CACAO CASHEW AND FRUITS

Preparation Time	Total Time	Yield
10 minutes	30 minutes	10 servings

INGREDIENTS

- 1/2 cup (50 g) shredded coconut, unsweetened
- 1/3 cup (40 g) raw cashew nuts, unsalted
- 1/4 cup (15 g) raw cacao powder
- 2 tablespoon (20 g) sunflower seeds
- 2 tablespoons (20 g) pumpkin seeds
- 1 teaspoon (2 g) ground cinnamon
- 1/2 cup (60 g) dried currants
- 1/2 cup (60 g) dried figs, coarsely chopped
- 1 cup (180 g) pitted fresh dates, coarsely chopped
- 2 tablespoons (30 ml) coconut oil, melted

PROCEDURE

- Combine the coconut, cashew nuts, cacao powder, sunflower seeds, pumpkin seeds, and cinnamon in your food processor. Process until everything are finely chopped.
- Add the currants and figs. Process again until combined well.
- With motor running, gradually add the dates, and then the coconut oil continue mixing until the mixture starts to come together.

- Using clean hands, bring the mixture together completely, add 1-2 teaspoons cold water, if needed.
- Press the mixture evenly into a 9-inch square baking tin, with the back of a metal spoon. Cover and refrigerate for a couple of hours before cutting into portions.
- Serve and enjoy!

NUTRITIONAL INFORMATION

Energy	Fat	Carbohydrates	Protein	Sodium
179 calories	7.9 g	26.7 g	3.2 g	8 mg

GLUTEN-FREE NUTTY GRANOLA BAR

Preparation Time	Total Time	Yield
10 minutes	40 minutes	12 servings

INGREDIENTS

- 1-1/2 cups (185 g) roasted whole almonds
- 1 cup (185 g) toasted quinoa
- 1/3 cup (60 g) chocolate chips
- 2 tablespoons (20 g) hemp seeds
- 2 tablespoons (20 g) sesame seeds, toasted
- 1 teaspoon (2 g) ground cinnamon
- 1/2 cup pitted fresh dates, finely chopped
- 1/2 cup (170 ml) honey
- 1/2 cup (125 g) cashew nut butter
- 1/4 cup (60 ml) coconut oil
- 1 teaspoon (5 ml) vanilla extract
- 2 oz. (60 g) dark chocolate, melted

PROCEDURE

- Grease a 9 x 13-inch baking pan and line base and 2 long sides with foil or baking paper.
- Place the almonds, quinoa, chocolate chips, hemp seeds, sesame seeds, cinnamon, and dates in a large bowl.
- Combine honey, cashew nut butter, coconut oil, and vanilla extract in a small saucepan. Cook, over low heat, stirring frequently until well combined and smooth.

- Stir in wet mixture into the dry ingredients. Mix thoroughly until evenly coated and blended.
- Using wet hands or a spatula, press the mixture firmly into the prepared pan. Cover and chill until set, about 1-2 hours. Once set, cut into 16 portions.
- Drizzle bars with melted chocolate if desired.
- Serve or store in an airtight container in the refrigerator for up to one week.

NUTRITIONAL INFORMATION

Energy	Fat	Carbohydrates	Protein	Sodium
206 calories	11.0 g	23.9 g	4.6 g	5 mg

CARDAMOM-SPICED QUINOA AND COCONUT BARS

Preparation Time	Total Time	Yield
10 minutes	40 minutes	16 servings

INGREDIENTS

- 2 cups (370 g) quinoa, slightly toasted
- 1 cup (100 g) shredded coconut, unsweetened
- 1/4 cup (25 g) almond meal
- 2 tablespoons (20 g) hemp seeds
- 1 teaspoon (2 g) ground cardamom
- 1/4 teaspoon (1.5 g) kosher salt
- 1/2 cup (125 g) applesauce, unsweetened
- 3/4 cup (240 ml) agave nectar
- 2 tablespoons (30 ml) coconut oil
- 1 teaspoon (5 ml) pure vanilla extract
- cooking oil spray

PROCEDURE

- Line a 9-inch square pan with aluminum foil. Lightly grease the foil with oil spray. Preheat and set your oven to 350 F (175 C).
- Mix together the quinoa, shredded coconut, almond meal, hemp seeds, cardamom, and salt in a medium bowl. Set aside.
- In a small bowl, whisk the applesauce, agave nectar, coconut oil, and vanilla extract to combine. Then, pour

this mixture into the bowl with the quinoa mixture. Mix until everything is coated well.

- With a piece of wax paper, press mixture firmly into the pan (so it won't stick to your fingers and to make an even layer at the bottom of the pan).
- Bake in the oven for about 20-25 minutes, or until it begins to turn golden brown. Take it out of the oven and allow to cool completely in the pan before cutting into portions.
- Store them in an airtight container, in between layers of wax paper, for up to one week inside the refrigerator.

NUTRITIONAL INFORMATION

Energy	Fat	Carbohydrates	Protein	Sodium
179 calories	6.3 g	27.8 g	4.1 g	37 mg

EASY PROTEIN BAR WITH HONEY

Preparation Time	Total Time	Yield
10 minutes	40 minutes	10 servings

INGREDIENTS

- 1/2 cup (90 g) pre-washed raw quinoa
- 1/2 cup (50 g) brown rice krispies
- 1 cup (125 g) dry roasted mixed nuts
- 1 cup (125 g) mixed dried fruits
- 1/2 cup (50 g) shredded coconut
- 2/3 cup (230 ml) honey
- 2 tablespoons (30 g) almond butter
- 1/2 teaspoon (2.5 g) salt
- 1/2 teaspoon (2.5 ml) pure vanilla extract
- cooking oil spray

PROCEDURE

- Line a 9-inch square pan with aluminum foil. Lightly grease the foil with oil spray. Preheat and set your oven to 350 F (175 C).
- Then, pop the quinoa in a large pan or skillet. Set aside to cool.
- Combine the mixed nuts and mixed fruits to a food processor. Process in short pulses, until coarsely chopped.
- Mix together the quinoa, brown rice krispies, shredded coconut, chopped nuts and fruits to a medium bowl. Set aside.

- Place the honey, almond butter, salt, and vanilla in a microwave-proof bowl or measuring cup. Microwave very briefly, until just heated. Pour this mixture into the bowl with the quinoa mixture. Mix until everything is coated well.
- With a piece of wax paper, press mixture firmly into the pan (so it won't stick to your fingers and to make an even layer at the bottom of the pan).
- Bake mixture in the oven for about 20-25 minutes, or until it begins to turn golden brown. Take it out of the oven and allow to cool completely in the pan before cutting into portions.
- Store them in an airtight container, in between layers of wax or baking paper, for up to one week inside the refrigerator.

NUTRITIONAL INFORMATION

Energy	Fat	Carbohydrates	Protein	Sodium
188 calories	6.7 g	31.7 g	3.3 g	80 mg

SPICED GRANOLA BAR WITH BANANA

Preparation Time	Total Time	Yield
10 minutes	40 minutes	12 servings

INGREDIENTS

- 2 (150 g) ripe bananas
- 1 teaspoon (5 ml) pure vanilla extract
- 1/4 cup (80 ml) agave nectar
- 2 tablespoons (30 g) applesauce, unsweetened
- 1/2 teaspoon (1 g) ground cinnamon
- 1/4 teaspoon (0.5 g) grated nutmeg
- 2 cups (200 g) rolled oats
- 1/2 teaspoon (2.5 g) kosher salt
- 1/3 cup (60 g) pitted dried dates, chopped
- 1/3 cup (35 g) pecan nuts, chopped
- 2 oz. (60 g) dark chocolate, melted
- cooking oil spray

PROCEDURE

- Preheat and set your oven to 350 F (175 C). Lightly grease a 9 x 9-inch square baking dish with oil spray.
- Peel the bananas and mash in a medium mixing bowl until smooth.
- Stir in the vanilla, agave nectar, applesauce, cinnamon, and nutmeg.
- Add the oats, salt, dates, and pecans. Mix well.
- Transfer and press the mixture firmly into the baking pan. Bake for 20-25 minutes or until the edges just

begin to turn golden. Remove from heat.

- Place the baking pan on a rack and let it cool completely before cutting into bars. Drizzle with melted chocolate.

- Serve and store leftover bars in an airtight container inside the refrigerator.

NUTRITIONAL INFORMATION

Energy	Fat	Carbohydrates	Protein	Sodium
150 calories	4.1 g	26.5 g	2.8 g	102 mg

CHOCO HAZELNUT POWER BAR

Preparation Time	Total Time	Yield
10 minutes	40 minutes	16 servings

INGREDIENTS

- 2/3 cup (220 ml) agave nectar
- 1/3 cup (85 g) smooth and creamy peanut butter
- 2 tablespoons (7 g) cocoa powder
- 2 tablespoons (30 ml) coconut oil
- 1 teaspoon (5 ml) pure vanilla extract
- 1 cup (100 g) oat flour
- 1 cup (100 g) rolled oats
- 1/2 cup (60 g) hazelnuts, chopped
- 1/2 cup (50 g) shredded coconut, unsweetened
- 2 tablespoons (20 g) flaxseeds
- 1/2 teaspoon (1 g) cinnamon, ground
- 1/4 teaspoon (1.5 g) kosher salt
- 1/3 cup (40 g) seedless raisins
- 1 tablespoon (10 g) sunflower seeds
- cooking oil spray

PROCEDURE

- Line a 9 x 13 baking dish with parchment paper or foil that has been lightly sprayed with oil, leaving an overhang on the sides for easy removal of bars.
- Combine the agave nectar, peanut butter, cocoa powder, coconut oil, and vanilla in a medium saucepan. Heat over medium-low flame until smooth,

about 1 minute. Remove from the heat.
- Add in the oat flour, rolled oats, hazelnuts, shredded coconut, flaxseeds, cinnamon, and salt. Mix to combine
- Stir in the raisins and sunflower seeds.
- Transfer and press the mixture evenly into the baking pan. Bake for 20-25 minutes.
- Place the baking pan on a wire rack and let it cool completely before cutting into bars.
- Serve and store leftover bars in an airtight container inside the refrigerator.

NUTRITIONAL INFORMATION

Energy	Fat	Carbohydrates	Protein	Sodium
177 calories	7.9 g	24.8 g	3.0 g	25 mg

ENERGY BAR WITH PISTACHIOS AND CRANBERRIES

Preparation Time	Total Time	Yield
10 minutes	40 minutes	12 servings

INGREDIENTS

- 2 cups (200 g) old-fashioned oats
- 1/2 cup (50 g) brown rice krispies
- 1/2 cup (60 g) pistachio nuts, coarsely chopped
- 1/2 cup (60 g) dried cranberries
- 1/4 cup (40 g) sesame seeds
- 1/4 teaspoon (1.5 g) kosher salt
- 1/2 cup (125 g) almond butter
- 1/4 cup (80 ml) maple syrup
- 1/4 cup (80 ml) agave nectar
- 1 teaspoon (5 ml) pure vanilla extract

PROCEDURE

- Preheat your oven to 350 F (175 C). Line a 9 x 13 baking pan with wax or parchment paper.
- In a large bowl place the oats, rice krispies, pistachio nuts, dried cranberries, sesame seeds, and salt. Mix together.
- In a small microwave safe bowl, mix together the almond butter, maple syrup, and agave nectar. Microwave briefly, until just heated and then stir in vanilla.

- Pour the almond butter mixture to the oat mixture and mix until everything is coated well. Transfer and press firmly into the prepared pan. Bake for 20–25 minutes. Take it out of the oven and allow to cool completely in the pan before cutting into portions.
- Serve or store in an airtight container.

NUTRITIONAL INFORMATION

Energy	Fat	Carbohydrates	Protein	Sodium
165 calories	7.4 g	23.0 g	3.8 g	95 mg

CHOCOLATE MACADAMIA POWER BAR

Preparation Time	Total Time	Yield
10 minutes	40 minutes	12 servings

INGREDIENTS

- 2-1/2 cups (250 g) rolled oats
- 1 cup (145 g) macadamia nuts, chopped
- 2/3 cup (120 g) semisweet chocolate chips
- 1/2 cup (125 g) applesauce, unsweetened
- 1/3 cup (110 ml) agave nectar
- 1 teaspoon (5 ml) vanilla extract
- 1/4 tsp. (1.5 g) Kosher salt
- cooking oil spray

PROCEDURE

- Preheat and set your oven to 350 F (175 C). Line a 9 x 13-inch baking dish or pan with foil or parchment paper and spray lightly with oil.
- Mix the oats and macadamia nuts together in a large bowl. Set aside.
- In a small saucepan, combine the chocolate chips, applesauce, agave nectar, vanilla, and salt. Heat over moderate flame until chocolate is melted. Remove from the heat.
- Pour the chocolate mixture into the bowl with oats. Mix until coated well.

- Press this mixture firmly into the prepared baking pan.
- Bake for about 20-25 minutes. Take it out of the oven and allow to cool completely in the pan before cutting into portions.
- Serve and enjoy.

NUTRITIONAL INFORMATION

Energy	Fat	Carbohydrates	Protein	Sodium
178 calories	9.9 g	21.7 g	2.4 g	36 mg

PROTEIN BAR DELIGHT

Preparation Time	Total Time	Yield
15 minutes	40 minutes	16 servings

INGREDIENTS

- 1 cup (185 g) pre-washed raw quinoa
- 1 cup (30 g) rice krispies
- 1 cup (100 g) old-fashioned oats, toasted
- 1/2 cup (60 g) dry roasted almonds, chopped
- 1/4 cup (40 g) pumpkin seeds
- 1/2 cup (160 ml) brown rice syrup
- 1/4 cup (60 g) almond butter
- 1/2 teaspoon (2.5 g) salt
- 6 oz. (180 g) semisweet chocolate chips, melted
- cooking oil spray

PROCEDURE

- Line a 9 x 13-inch baking dish with aluminum foil or wax paper. Lightly grease the foil with oil spray.
- Then, pop the quinoa in a large pan or skillet. Set aside to cool.
- Mix together the quinoa, rice krispies, oats, almonds, and pumpkin seeds in a medium bowl. Set aside.
- Place the brown rice syrup, almond butter, and salt in a small saucepan. Cook, stirring over low flame for about 5 minutes, or until heated through. Pour this mixture into the bowl with the quinoa mixture. Mix until everything is coated well.
- Pour the melted chocolate and spread to make an even layer at the bottom of the pan. Then, top with the

quinoa mixture. With a piece of wax paper, press the mixture firmly into the pan.

- Chill in the refrigerator for at least an hour before cutting into bars.
- Serve or store them in an airtight container.

NUTRITIONAL INFORMATION

Energy	Fat	Carbohydrates	Protein	Sodium
157 calories	5.6 g	27.4 g	4.5 g	91 mg

GRANOLA BAR WITH WALNUT AND RAISIN

Preparation Time	Total Time	Yield
10 minutes	40 minutes	16 servings

INGREDIENTS

- 2 cups (200 g) old-fashioned oats
- 1 cup (100 g) walnuts, chopped
- 2 tablespoons (15 g) wheat germ
- 1/2 cup (60 g) dried raisins
- 1/2 cup (160 ml) honey
- 1/4 cup (60 g) applesauce, unsweetened, add more if needed
- 1/2 teaspoon (2.5 g) kosher salt
- 1 teaspoon (5 ml) pure vanilla extract
- cooking oil spray

PROCEDURE

- Line a 9-inch square pan with aluminum foil. Lightly grease the foil with oil spray. Preheat and set your oven to 325 F (160 C).
- Mix together the oats, walnuts, wheat germ, and raisins in a large bowl.
- Stir in honey, applesauce, salt, and vanilla until combined and coated well.
- With a piece of wax paper, press mixture firmly into the pan.
- Bake in the oven for about 20-25 minutes, or until it begins to turn golden brown. Take it out of the oven

and allow to cool completely in the pan before cutting into portions.

- Store them in an airtight container, in between layers of wax or parchment paper, for up to one week inside the refrigerator.

NUTRITIONAL INFORMATION

Energy	Fat	Carbohydrates	Protein	Sodium
179 calories	6.0 g	27.8 g	4.8 g	75 mg

QUINOA CHIA AND SESAME BAR

Preparation Time	Total Time	Yield
10 minutes	40 minutes	12 servings

INGREDIENTS

- 1-½ cups (150 g) old-fashioned oats
- 1 cup (125 g) raw almonds
- 1/3 cup (60 g) chia seeds
- 1/3 cup (60 g) sesame seeds
- 2/3 cup (230 ml) honey
- 1/3 cup (85 g) almond butter, add more if needed

PROCEDURE

- Preheat and set your oven to 300 F (150 C).
- Place the oat and almond mixture in a food processor and process until finely ground. Transfer to a medium bowl.
- Add the chia seeds and sesame seeds.
- Warm the honey and almond butter in a small saucepan over low heat. Pour over oat mixture and then mix until coated well.
- Transfer to an 8 x 8-inch baking pan lined with parchment paper so they can be lifted out easily.
- Flatten mixture with a spatula to get them tightly packed and prevent from being crumbly.
- Bake for about 20 minutes. Take it out of the oven and allow to cool completely in the pan before cutting into portions.

- Serve or store in an airtight container for up to a week inside the refrigerator or freezer, if not eating right away.

NUTRITIONAL INFORMATION

Energy	Fat	Carbohydrates	Protein	Sodium
177 calories	8.2 g	24.7 g	4.2 g	20 mg

OAT AND COCONUT ENERGY BAR WITH CASHEW

Preparation Time	Total Time	Yield
10 minutes	40 minutes	16 servings

INGREDIENTS

- 2 cups (200 g) rolled oats
- 1 cup (100 g) shredded coconut, unsweetened
- 1 cup (125 g) cashew nuts, chopped
- 1 (60 g) whole egg, lightly beaten
- 3/4 cup (240 g) agave nectar
- 1/4 cup (60 g) applesauce, unsweetened
- cooking oil spray

PROCEDURE

- Line a 9-inch square pan with aluminum foil. Grease the foil lightly with oil spray. Preheat and set your oven to 350 F (175 C).
- Mix together the oats, shredded coconut, and cashews in a medium bowl. Make a well in the center.
- Add the egg, agave nectar, and applesauce. Mix to combine well.
- Pour this mixture into the prepared baking pan. Smoothen and press the top using a spatula.
- Bake for about 25-30 minutes, or until it begins to turn golden brown. Take it out of the oven and allow to cool completely in the pan before cutting into portions.

- Serve or store them in an airtight container, in between layers of wax or parchment paper, for up to one week inside the refrigerator.

NUTRITIONAL INFORMATION

Energy	Fat	Carbohydrates	Protein	Sodium
189 calories	10.0 g	24.2 g	3.1 g	9 mg

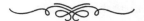

PUMPKIN BARS WITH PECANS

Preparation Time	Total Time	Yield
10 minutes	1 hour	24 servings

INGREDIENTS

- 1-1/4 cup (160 g) all-purpose flour
- 2/3 cup (70 g) old-fashioned oats
- 2/3 cup (150 g) brown sugar, packed
- 1/2 cup (125 g) butter, softened
- 1/2 cup (160 ml) agave nectar
- 1/4 cup (80 ml) maple syrup
- 2 cups (500 g) pumpkin puree
- 1 can (350 ml) evaporated Milk
- 2 (60 g) whole eggs
- 2 teaspoons (4 g) pumpkin pie spice
- 2/3 cup (70 g) pecan nuts, chopped
- 1/4 cup (55 g) packed brown sugar
- cooking oil spray

PROCEDURE

- Preheat and set your oven to 350 F (175 C).
- Combine the flour, oats, brown sugar, and butter in small mixer bowl. Beat at low speed for about 2 minutes, or until crumbly. Press at the bottom of ungreased 13 x 9-inch baking dish.
- Bake in the oven for 10 minutes.
- Mix together the agave nectar, maple syrup, pumpkin puree, evaporated milk, eggs, and the pumpkin pie

spice in large mixer bowl. Beat at medium speed for about 2-3 minutes. Pour this mixture over crust. Bake for 20 minutes.

- Place the pecans and brown sugar in small bowl. Mix well.
- Sprinkle pecan topping over filling. Continue baking for another 10 minutes, or until tested done. Take it out of the oven and allow to cool completely in the pan before cutting into portions.
- Serve or store in an airtight container inside the refrigerator.

NUTRITIONAL INFORMATION

Energy	Fat	Carbohydrates	Protein	Sodium
165 calories	7.7 g	21.9 g	3.2 g	52 mg

CHUNKY GRANOLA BAR

Preparation Time	Total Time	Yield
10 minutes	40 minutes	12 servings

INGREDIENTS

- 1 cup (100 g) rolled oats, toasted
- 1 cup (125 g) dry roasted almonds, coarsely chopped
- 1/2 cup (90 g) pitted dates, coarsely chopped
- 1/4 cup (30 g) dried cherries
- 1/4 cup (40 g) sunflower seeds
- 1/4 cup (40 g) pumpkin seeds
- 2 tablespoons (20 g) flaxseeds
- 2 tablespoons (20 g) hemp seeds
- 1 teaspoon (2 g) ground cinnamon
- 1/3 cup (85 g) applesauce, unsweetened, add more if needed
- 1/3 cup (110 ml) agave nectar

PROCEDURE

- Preheat and set your oven to 350 F (175 C). Line a 9 x 13 baking pan with wax or parchment paper.
- In a large bowl place the oats, almonds, dates, dried cherries, sunflower seeds, pumpkin seeds, flaxseeds, hemp seeds, and cinnamon. Mix to combine well.
- Stir in applesauce and agave nectar. Pour this mixture into the oat mixture and mix until everything is coated well.
- With a piece of wax paper, press mixture firmly into the pan. Bake for 20-25 minutes. Take it out of the oven and allow to cool completely in the pan before cutting

into portions.

- Serve or store in airtight container.

NUTRITIONAL INFORMATION

Energy	Fat	Carbohydrates	Protein	Sodium
171 calories	7.8 g	22.7 g	4.7 g	52 mg

PEANUT BUTTER AND QUINOA PROTEIN BAR

Preparation Time	Total Time	Yield
10 minutes	40 minutes	16 servings

INGREDIENTS

- 1-1/2 cups (180 g) pre-washed raw quinoa
- 2/3 cup (130 g) raw amaranth
- 1/2 cup (50 g) shredded coconut, unsweetened
- 1/2 cup (160 ml) brown rice syrup
- 1/2 cup (125 g) peanut butter
- 1-1/2 teaspoon (3 g) ground cinnamon
- 1/2 teaspoon (2.5 g) kosher salt
- 1 teaspoon (5 ml) pure vanilla extract
- cooking oil spray

PROCEDURE

- Line a 9-inch square pan with parchment paper or aluminum foil and lightly grease with oil spray. Preheat and set your oven to 350 F (175 C).
- Then, pop the quinoa and amaranth in a large pan or skillet. Transfer to a mixing bowl and allow the mixture to cool.
- Combine the brown rice syrup, peanut butter, cinnamon, and salt in a small saucepan. Cook over moderate flame until heated through and peanut butter is melted. Stir in vanilla extract. Pour this mixture into the bowl with the quinoa mixture. Mix until everything is coated well.

- With a piece of wax paper, press mixture firmly into the pan.
- Bake in the oven for about 20-25 minutes, or until it begins to turn golden brown. Take it out of the oven and allow to cool completely in the pan before cutting into portions.
- Serve or store them in an airtight container, in between layers of wax paper, for up to one week inside the refrigerator.

NUTRITIONAL INFORMATION

Energy	Fat	Carbohydrates	Protein	Sodium
174 calories	6.4 g	25.5 g	5.8 g	121 mg

DATE OAT AND FLAX POWER BAR

Preparation Time	Total Time	Yield
15 minutes	45 minutes	12 servings

INGREDIENTS

Homemade Date Paste

- 2 cups (360 g) pitted Medjool dates
- 1/2 cup (125 ml) water

Granola Bars

- 1/4 cup (60 g) almond butter
- 2 tablespoons (30 ml) coconut oil
- 1 teaspoon (5 ml) pure vanilla extract
- 2-1/2 cups (250 g) old-fashioned oats, toasted
- 1/2 cup (80 g) flaxseeds
- 1/2 teaspoon (1 g) ground cinnamon
- 1/4 teaspoon (0.5 g) nutmeg
- 1/4 teaspoon (1.5 g) kosher salt
- cooking oil spray

PROCEDURE

- Line a 9 x 13-inch baking pan with parchment paper or foil that has been sprayed lightly with oil leaving an overhang on the sides of the pan for easy removal.
- Put the dates and water to a medium saucepan and cook on medium low heat. Using a fork, mash the dates as the mixture heats up, stirring frequently. The dates will soften after about 5 minutes. Continue

stirring and mashing until it forms a thick paste, it is fine to have some bits.

- Stir in almond butter, coconut oil, and vanilla. Turn off the heat.
- Add in the oats, flaxseeds, cinnamon, nutmeg, and salt. Mix until coated well.
- Transfer into the prepared pan. Press using a sheet of parchment paper to make a firm and even layer. Cover and chill before cutting into portions.
- Serve or store in airtight container inside the refrigerator for up to one week.

NUTRITIONAL INFORMATION

Energy	Fat	Carbohydrates	Protein	Sodium
164 calories	5.2 g	26.8 g	3.7 g	52 mg

ALMOND CRANBERRY ENERGY BAR WITH HONEY

Preparation Time	Total Time	Yield
10 minutes	40 minutes	12 servings

INGREDIENTS

- 2 cups (200 g) rolled oats, ground
- 1 cup (125 g) almonds, chopped
- 1/2 cup (60 g) dried cranberries
- 1/2 cup (125 g) applesauce, unsweetened
- 1/2 cup (160 g) honey
- 1 teaspoon (5 ml) vanilla extract
- 1/4 tsp. (1.5 g) Kosher salt
- cooking oil spray

PROCEDURE

- Preheat and set your oven to 350 F (175 C). Line a 9 x 13-inch baking dish or pan with foil or parchment paper and spray lightly with oil.
- Mix the oats, almonds, dried cranberries, applesauce, honey, vanilla extract, and salt together in a large bowl.
- Press the energy bar mixture firmly into the prepared baking pan.
- Bake for about 20-25 minutes. Take it out of the oven and allow to cool completely in the pan before cutting into portions.

- Serve and enjoy.

NUTRITIONAL INFORMATION

Energy	Fat	Carbohydrates	Protein	Sodium
184 calories	4.9 g	24.2 g	3.5 g	52 mg

THE ULTIMATE ENERGY BAR

Preparation Time	Total Time	Yield
15 minutes	45 minutes	12 servings

INGREDIENTS

- 2 tablespoons (30 ml) coconut oil
- 1/2 cup (125 g) almond butter
- 1/4 cup (60 g) mashed banana
- 1/4 cup (80 ml) brown rice syrup
- 1 teaspoon (2 g) ground cinnamon
- 1 teaspoon (5 ml) pure vanilla extract
- 2 cups (200 g) old fashioned oats
- 3/4 cup (90 g) almonds, coarsely chopped
- 3/4 cup (75 g) pecan nuts, coarsely chopped
- 1/2 cup (60 g) sultanas
- 1/2 cup (60 g) dried apricots

PROCEDURE

- Preheat and set your oven to 300 F (150 C).
- In a small saucepan over medium-low heat, heat the coconut oil and then stir in almond butter until combined well.
- Add the mashed banana, brown rice syrup, cinnamon, and vanilla extract. Mix well and remove from heat.
- In a heat-proof glass bowl, mix together the oats, almonds, pecans, sultanas, and apricots.
- Stir in almond butter mixture until coated well.
- Transfer the mixture into a baking pan and spread out

the granola evenly. Using a parchment paper press it down to make firm bars.
- Bake for about 25–30 minutes. Take it out of the oven and allow to cool completely in the pan before cutting into portions.
- Serve or store in an airtight container.

NUTRITIONAL INFORMATION

Energy	Fat	Carbohydrates	Protein	Sodium
179 calories	10.1 g	20.7 g	4.1 g	6 mg

CHEWY ENERGY BAR

Preparation Time	Total Time	Yield
10 minutes	40 minutes	24 servings

INGREDIENTS

- 3 cups (300 g) quick cooking oats
- 1 cup (100 g) almond flour
- 2/3 cup (70 g) sweetened coconut flakes
- 1 cup (125 g) mixed dried fruits, chopped
- 2 teaspoons (4 g) ground cinnamon
- 1 teaspoon (6 g) baking soda
- 1 cup (250 g) applesauce, unsweetened
- 1/3 cup (85 g) melted butter, cooled
- 2/3 cup (230 ml) honey
- 1 (60 g) whole egg

PROCEDURE

- Preheat and set your oven to 350 F (175 C).
- Combine the oats, almond flour, coconut flakes, mixed dried fruits, cinnamon, and baking soda in large mixing bowl.
- In separate bowl, mix together the applesauce, melted butter, honey, and egg. Then, pour this mixture into the bowl with dry ingredients. Mix until combined well. Spread and press the mixture evenly into a lightly greased 9 x 13-inch baking pan.
- Bake for 20-25 minutes, or until lightly browned. Take it out of the oven and allow to cool completely in the pan before cutting into portions.
- Serve or store in an airtight container.

NUTRITIONAL INFORMATION

Energy	Fat	Carbohydrates	Protein	Sodium
184 calories	9.0 g	25.1 g	2.8 g	78 mg

CHOCO WALNUT AND APRICOT BAR

Preparation Time	Total Time	Yield
10 minutes	40 minutes	12 servings

INGREDIENTS

- 1 cup (100 g) old-fashioned oats
- 1 cup (100 g) walnuts
- 1 cup (125 g) dried apricots, chopped
- 1/2 cup (160 ml) agave nectar
- 1/4 cup (60 g) unsweetened applesauce, add more if needed
- 1/2 teaspoon (2.5 g) kosher salt
- 1 teaspoon (5 ml) pure vanilla extract
- cooking oil spray

PROCEDURE

- Line a 9 x 13-inch baking pan with parchment paper or aluminum foil and lightly grease with oil spray. Preheat and set your oven to 325 F (160 C).
- Mix together the oats, walnuts, and apricots in a large bowl.
- Stir in agave nectar, applesauce, salt, and vanilla extract until coated well.
- With a piece of wax paper, press the mixture firmly into the pan.
- Bake in the oven for about 20-25 minutes, or until it begins to turn golden brown. Take it out of the oven and allow to cool completely in the pan before cutting

into portions.

- Serve or store them in an airtight container, in between layers of parchment paper, for up to one week inside the refrigerator.

NUTRITIONAL INFORMATION

Energy	Fat	Carbohydrates	Protein	Sodium
159 calories	6.7 g	23.7 g	3.8 g	99 mg

BUCKWHEAT PISTACHIO AND CURRANT BAR

Preparation Time	Total Time	Yield
30 minutes	1 hours 30 minutes	20 servings

INGREDIENTS

- 2 cups (200 g) old-fashioned rolled oats, toasted
- 1 cup (170 g) buckwheat groats, toasted
- 1 cup (125 g) dried currants
- 1/2 cup (60 g) pistachio nuts, chopped
- 1/2 cup (30 g) puffed millet
- 1/4 cup (40 g) hemp seeds
- 1/4 cup (40 g) chia seeds
- 1 teaspoon (2 g) cinnamon
- 1/4 teaspoon (0.5 g) cardamom
- 2/3 cup (165 g) almond butter
- 2/3 cup (220 ml) brown rice syrup
- 1/2 cup (125 ml) coconut oil
- 2 teaspoons (10 ml) pure vanilla extract
- 1/4 teaspoon (0.5 g) kosher salt

PROCEDURE

- In a large bowl, mix together the oats, buckwheat groats, dried currants, pistachios, puffed millet, hemp seeds, chia seeds, cinnamon, and cardamom.
- Combine the almond butter, brown rice syrup, coconut oil, vanilla extract, and salt in a small saucepan over

low heat until melted and blended thoroughly. Pour this warm mixture into the bowl with dry ingredients and mix until coated well.

- Line a medium-sized jelly roll pan with foil or parchment paper, just make sure you have edges of foil sticking up on all sides.
- Pour the energy bar mixture into the pan and press it down with a spatula to create an even layer.
- Place the pan in the freezer for at least 2 hours to set before cutting into bars.
- Serve or store in an airtight container in the refrigerator or freezer.

NUTRITIONAL INFORMATION

Energy	Fat	Carbohydrates	Protein	Sodium
175 calories	9.6 g	19.1 g	3.6 g	46 mg

PEANUT AND CEREAL BAR

Preparation Time	Total Time	Yield
10 minutes	40 minutes	12 servings

INGREDIENTS

- 1 cup (250 g) peanut butter
- 1/2 cup (110 g) brown sugar
- 1-1/4 cups (125 g) old-fashioned rolled oats, ground
- 1/2 cup (50 g) wheat germ
- 1/4 cup (25 g) shredded coconut, unsweetened
- 1/4 cup (40 g) peanuts, chopped
- 1/4 cup (40 g) flaxseeds, ground
- cooking oil spray

PROCEDURE

- Preheat and set your oven to 325 F (160 C). Grease a 9 x 13-inch baking pan with oil spray and line with baking paper.
- In a small saucepan, melt the peanut butter with brown sugar until smooth.
- Place the oats, wheat germ, shredded coconut, peanuts, and ground flaxseeds in a large bowl. Add the peanut butter mixture. Mix until coated well.
- Press mixture into the prepared baking pan to make firm bars.
- Bake for 20-25 minutes. Take it out of the oven and allow to cool completely in the pan before cutting into portions.

- Serve or store in an airtight container.

NUTRITIONAL INFORMATION

Energy	Fat	Carbohydrates	Protein	Sodium
190 calories	12.0 g	16.3 g	6.8 g	70 mg

RECIPE INDEX

G

Gluten-Free Carrot and Raisin Power Bar 12
Gluten-Free Nutty Granola Bar 66
Granola Bar with Dried Fruits 40
Granola Bar with Pomegranate 44
Granola Bar with Walnut and Raisin 82
Granola with Raspberry and Pecan 32

M

Mixed Fruit Muesli Bar 62
Muesli Bar with Chocolate Chips and Almonds 38

N

No-Bake Apricot and Sultana Protein Bars 54
Nutty Energy Bars with Sunflower Seeds 60

O

Oat and Coconut Energy Bar with Cashew 86

P

Peanut and Cereal Bar 106
Peanut Butter and Quinoa Protein Bar 92
Peanut Butter Energy Bars 58
Power Bar with Cacao Cashew and Fruits 64
Power Bar with Strawberries 18
Power-Packed Cereal Bar 28
Protein Bar Delight 80
Pumpkin Bars with Pecans 88

Q

Quinoa Chia and Sesame Bar 84

R

Raw Vegan Energy Bar with Cacao 20

S

Spiced Granola Bar with Banana 72
Strawberry Filled Energy Bars 34

We want to thank you for purchasing this book. Our writers and creative team took pride in creating this book, and we have tried to make it as enjoyable as possible.

We would love to hear from you, kindly leave a review if you enjoyed this book so we can do more. Your reviews on our books are highly appreciated. Also, if you have any comments or suggestions, you may reach us at

info@contentarcade.com

Regards,
Content Arcade Publishing Team

Made in United States
Troutdale, OR
11/20/2024

25101646R00070